Mindfulness

Live in the Moment

by

Dharma Hazari

Disclaimer

No part of this publication may be reproduced or transmitted in any form or by any means, mechanical or electronic, including photocopying or recording, or by any information storage and retrieval system, or transmitted by email without permission in writing from the publisher.

While all attempts have been made to verify the information provided in this publication, neither the author nor the publisher assumes any responsibility for errors, omissions, or contrary interpretations of the subject matter herein.

This book is for entertainment purposes only. The views expressed are those of the author alone, and should not be taken as expert instruction or commands. The reader is responsible for his or her own actions.

Adherence to all applicable laws and regulations, including international, federal, state, and local governing professional licensing, business practices, advertising, and all other aspects of doing business in the US, Canada, or any other jurisdiction is the sole responsibility of the purchaser or reader.

Neither the author nor the publisher assumes any responsibility or liability whatsoever on the behalf of the purchaser or reader of these materials.

Any perceived slight of any individual or organization is purely unintentional.

What is this about ?

Greetings and welcome to this book on Mindfulness. My name is Dharma Hazari. I have written this book to share some insights on what mindfulness is, how it can help you and why it is crucial for your growth and well-being. Mindfulness is simply the act of being mindful about things in life. But there's more to it than that. And more importantly, it has huge upsides in terms of relieving stress, developing focus, inner peace and much more. Now let me share with you my own personal experiences on this subject.

My Journey with Mindfulness

Growing up in India, I've been bombarded with lots of ideas on yoga, meditation(dhyanam), buddhism, hinduism, spirituality etc. I started with yoga so that I can increase my flexibility and live a healthier lifestyle. That led me to meditation and mindfulness. My yoga teacher taught me the basics and gave me references to study further. So I did. Why? Because I was fascinated by the concept. And initially I wanted to build focus so I could do my class assignments faster. That would give me more time to play, have fun and pursue my other hobbies.

But as I started learning more, I realized that many religions and books stressed the importance of mindfulness. It was at the core of almost all practices that led to a better life. And that was being reflected in my own life. Not only did I build better focus but I was a much calmer being as a result. There was this shift in my personality and people were recognizing it. Although the change was more or less gradual, my friends and family would still be amazed at the transformation I managed to pull off. I had control over my mind like never before. All of this is not to brag but an honest attempt to convey to you the gravity and power of these methods.

That's my journey with mindfulness so far. It has been over 7 years since I took up this lifestyle and my results have been outstanding to say the least. So this book is my personal take on Mindfulness with some knowledge-nuggets I've picked up from other gurus and scientific research. For more valuable knowledge, meditation guides and more, join us at the link below.
http://bit.ly/spirituality-and-stuff

<u>Warning!</u>

If you feel like you are stuck in a negative cycle of bad behaviors or habits then you MUST read this book immediately. Do not wait. Do not postpone for later. It has been designed as a quick and compact read for this purpose. As you'll see in chapter-1, mindfulness has been proven through scientific research to better your life in countless ways. You can cut down future medical and shrink bills by developing the habit of mindfulness. So do yourself a favor and read all the chapters till the end. Takes notes if you need to. And don't forget – the most impactful thing this book can do is make you take action and develop the habit of mindfulness. Good Luck and let's begin.

Table of Contents

Chapter 1

Mindfulness - A Brief Introduction

So what is Mindfulness?

A simple definition is that mindfulness is the practice of being mindful. What is being mindful? It is a state of mind in which your attention is completely on the present moment and not diluted by distractions. It is categorized as an awareness of our surroundings and our actions.

The more aware you are, the more mindful you are. In general, mindfulness involves being aware of your thoughts, feelings, body sensations and surrounding environment. Since these are what the "present moment" comprises of.

Mindfulness is a process so it has a *subject* and an *object*. The *subject* is you because you are performing the act of mindfulness. The *object* is what you're being mindful of. There are two classes of *objects* you can be mindful of– the inside and the outside.

<u>The Inside</u> : Your thoughts, opinions about yourself and others, emotions, memories etc.

<u>The Outside</u> : Your skin, feet, arms, body parts, the ground you're sitting on, the objects nearby etc.

So mindfulness can essentially be defined as the awareness of the inside and the outside. One thing to note here is that when mindfulness is performed correctly, reality is perceived with complete clarity and no filters or biases. Proper mindfulness is seeing things as they are.

Also please note that mindfulness and meditation go hand in hand in many aspects. So in this book, they will often be used interchangeably based on the context.

Why should I do it ?

You should take up and practice mindfulness because there are tons of advantages to it. More of this will be covered in chapter-2. But here are some reasons why you should not delay any further in taking up mindfulness as a daily habit.

* Mindfulness is Medicine.

It has been shown that mindfulness helps people sleep better. So if you are someone who wants to have more sound sleep in your life, or feel exhausted very often then this is something you should definitely take up. It also reduces critical pains in your body like neck ache, back pain, arthritis, frequent headaches etc.

* Mindfulness increases your mental powers.

Neuroscientists from all over the world have published research which indicates that mindfulness training improves your ability to focus on demanding tasks. It also helps you ignore distractions better which also leads to increased focus and attention.

* Mindfulness helps you overcome addictions.

All of us have some form of addictions. Be it alcohol, cigarettes, junk food, drugs, talking, TV, social media etc. Over the years, mindfulness has been constantly found to help people fight and overcome addiction. This is because people who practice meditation can delay gratification and not react impulsively to triggers and cravings.

* Mindfulness actually makes you a calmer person.

Whenever we are in a stressful situation, our body releases a hormone called Cortisol which regulates the metabolism and suppresses our immune system. Recent studies have shown that people who practice mindfulness for 10-20 minutes daily have 40% lesser stress and anxiety. This is because mindfulness can lower the levels of cortisol in the body resulting in a calmer mind.

Where did this come from ?

Although there is no concrete evidence of the origin of mindfulness, it is rumored to have started around 15th century

BC in Indian Hinduism. Brahmin culture (caste of Hinduism) involved a lot of learning and reciting of scriptures and texts. In order to perform this heavy mental feat, the Brahmins had to free their thoughts up and develop concentration. They developed practices and principles for achieving this state. These later found their way into yoga and meditation which originated and spread across India. Mindfulness has traditionally been a fundamental underlying concept of Meditation.

After Buddhism came into existence and adopted some of the principles of yoga and meditation, it defined the concept of *Satipatthana* which basically means contemplation of body, feelings, mind and principles.

There are a lot of people who are responsible for the current widespread knowledge and interest in mindfulness across the globe. But more specifically, it was Thich Nhat Hanh who inspired the initial movement of practicing Buddhism in the west. And in the late 70's, Jon Kabat-Zinn, who is referred to as the founder of modern day mindfulness, developed a programme called Mindfulness Based Stress Reduction (MBSR) which became very popular and has helped people with various physical and mental conditions.

How do I achieve Mindfulness?

Details about practical techniques for mindfulness and integrating it into your day-to-day life are covered in chapters 3 and 4. But here's a simple method to get you started.

Find a quiet place and sit in a comfortable position. Take a few deep breaths and close your eyes. Now just relax and observe your breath first. Take note as the air comes in and goes out of your body. After a few minutes, extend your awareness of the present moment to the sounds, sensations, your wandering thoughts etc. Your sole job is to be a passive observer. Sounds easy but very difficult in the beginning. Try to be as detached to your thoughts as possible.

If you keep doing this particular activity for 10mins everyday, you will get more confident and calm. Later you can expand it to other areas and activities of your life. Eventually you can try to be present in the moment throughout your waking hours. That is the goal of mindfulness and meditation – to align your mind with true reality. Now let's take a look at what the scientists are saying on this matter.

Leading Research on Mindfulness.

With growing global interest on mindfulness and meditation, the amount of research conducted on the science behind it is also increasing.

- A study published in NeuroReport 2005 showed thicker cortical regions related to attention and sensory processing in long-term meditation practitioners compared to non-meditators. This means you will be less likely to loose your analytical and thinking abilities as you get older.

- Approximately 8 out of 10 people in the United States will experience lower back pain in their lives. In a study published in Journal of the American Medical

Association, researchers found that participants using Mindfulness based Stress Reduction (MBSR) programme had greater improvement in terms of back-pain as compared to the group in standard care.

- Brain studies on advanced meditators showed more activation in the areas that detect emotional cues, indicating more empathy and emotional intelligence.

- Another study published in Psychosomatic Medicine showed evidence that the body's immune system would react more robustly in antibody production after meditation training. Antibodies are proteins produced by the body to fight against various viruses, bacteria and other chemicals and defend the body from infection and disease.

- In a 2015 Central Michigan University study by Professor Adam Lueke, listening to mindfulness audio showed a decrease in implicit race and age bias.

References and Further Reading

http://marc.ucla.edu/

https://www.ncbi.nlm.nih.gov/pubmed/12883106

http://spp.sagepub.com/content/6/3/284

http://eomega.org

http://bemindful.co.uk/evidence-research/

http://mindfulschools.org

Chapter 2

Benefits of Mindfulness

The essence of mindfulness is to live in the present. With the advent of modern technology and social-media platforms, it has become hard to do just that – to forget all worries and live in the moment. Getting distracted has been made so easy for us. It's almost unfair. But if you are an ambitious person involved in the hustle and bustle of city life or if you just like to relax and have more peace of mind, mindfulness holds the key. Books like *The Power of Now* by Eckhart Tolle and *The Miracle of Mindfulnes* have been written in an attempt to help people achieve a higher sense of well-being through mindfulness. Without further ado, here are some practical benefits of mindfulness.

Benefit #1 : Self Awareness

The dictionary defines Self-awareness (noun) as : conscious knowledge of one's own character and feelings.

Business and Marketing guru, Gary Vaynerchuk says that self-awareness is your most important attribute. In his #AskGaryVee show on Youtube, he points out that self-awareness isn't just about betting on your strengths but also about accepting your short-comings i.e, to look at both sides of the coin. To see and accept things as they are in reality. This is probably one of the most immediate benefits you can get from mindfulness and meditation.

Awareness is transformative in and of itself.

\- Ken Wilber

When you practice mindfulness meditation, you become a passive observer. You detach yourself from all the thoughts and emotions you have. This develops a third-person perspective where you watch yourself from an objective viewpoint. And that has immense benefits when it comes to self-awareness and self-improvement.

Now, you might jump the gun here and assume that you're already pretty self-aware in your day-to-day activities. If you really are, that's great. But if you're doubtful about it, here's an example to measure your scale of awareness against.

Jack Murphy is a part-time shop assistant at a retail store in Ireland. Between his study, work, family, exercise and sleep he gets less than 2 hours to unwind and spend time with himself. His life was pretty hectic until he got into a sideways car accident. Although he survived it without major damage, it will be one of those unforgettable experiences for him. As most people who have been in an accident will tell you, time seems to slow down when you're in an accident, however short that might be. This is not because of providence or some kind of magic. If the laws of science don't change when you're in an accident then what does? Why does time slow down?

The answer is your level of awareness. This is a scientifically recorded phenomenon called *Slow Motion Perception* where your perceived time is longer because of your heightened awareness and richness of experience. According to Steve Taylor, a psychology lecturer at LMU, although clock time may be measured in minutes and hours, real time is perceived via experiences and how densely they're packed in our memory.

One of the most exciting and positive results of self-awareness is the richness of the experience. You forget everything else and get totally immersed in the moment. It's a bit hard to explain the magic of it unless you actually go through the experience of total self-awareness. But you don't have to get into a car accident to appreciate the importance of self-awareness. You can just start paying attention to your current surroundings and with enough practice of mindfulness, you can really become more self-aware and achieve a higher state of consciousness.

Benefit #2 : Stress-Reduction

Contrary to popular belief, stress is a normal part of life. And in certain scenarios, it can actually motivate and give us that extra push. But uncontrolled negative stress can lead to various issues with health and relationships. So it's safe to say that handling stress is a crucial skill that you need to learn if you want to live a balanced and happy life.

More information on how to handle and reduce stress can be found in chapter-7.

In dealing with stress, mindfulness is useful in two ways. The first is to reduce the level of stress by lowering the frequency of your mental vibrations. The second is to prevent you from entering stressful states of mind in the first place.

When you're mindful of your thoughts and emotions, it presents you with a subtle choice of stepping back and letting them play themselves out. By not taking them seriously, you are less likely to initiate the stress response. The mindfulness exercises described in chapter-3 will help you with this.

One of the major causes of stress in relationships is the inability to communicate emotions properly. As pointed out in the *leading-research* section of chapter-1, mindfulness can elevate your empathy levels and emotional intelligence over a period of time. With higher sensitivity and understanding of others' feelings, your relationships are bound to be more successful.

Benefit #3 : Increased Focus

There are numerous advantages to having increased focus levels. If you are a programmer it helps you find issues faster, write better code. If you are a student preparing for exams, it helps you have elongated study sessions with undisturbed concentration. If you are an artist, it helps you get into the "flow" state and produce magnificent artwork. It is quite common for mindfulness and meditation practitioners to experience a boost in their productivity.

Here's an insight. Getting distracted is possibly the number one reason for your lack of sustained focus. I guarantee that if you can manage to work with absolutely no distractions on your mind, your performance and productivity will skyrocket. In the 2006 drama film *Peaceful Warrior*, this exact lesson is taught by the teacher to the student using the phrase *"Take out the trash,*

Dan." The word *trash* is used figuratively here to represent all the irrelevant mental junk and distractions that stop us from achieving our peak focus.

Mindfulness helps in fighting distractions because your mind will be trained to stay in the present moment instead of ruminating about the past or future. Whenever you get distracted, you break away from experiencing the current moment. This can take some time but if you practice mindfulness regularly, your general life experiences will be much more streamlined with reality and you will gain the power to fend off distractions by staying in the moment.

Benefit #4 : Emotional Stability

In one research experiment, the fMRI data of participants from the mindfulness group indicated that they had lesser neural reactivity when exposed to sad films than the other group. This suggests that people who practice mindfulness can experience emotions selectively, choosing to be less reactive towards negative emotions such as sadness, depression, fear, anger, hatred etc. This is a sign of emotional maturity. It will help a lot if you're a sensitive person who finds it difficult to deal with haters, critics and negative feedback in general.

It's true how people say that you don't have control over what happens in life but only over how you react to it. And that's where mindfulness comes in. It can help you take hold of the proverbial "reins" of your monkey mind and let yourself feel the way you want to feel or not at all. Either way, you hold the wheel. You have the control.

Benefit #5 : Better Health

Over the years, increasing number of scientific studies have shown that mindfulness can lead to better overall health. Lower-back pain has been one of the most common issues people face, especially so for the last couple of decades due to the advent of computers and desk-jobs. In 2016, a Seattle-based research has found that people who take part in MBSR (Mindfulness-based Stress Reduction) which is a mix of meditation, yoga and body-awareness, had better results with various medical treatments when it came to back pain relief. So by developing a habit of mindfulness, you can expect to have higher energy levels, increased quality of sleep, faster recovery from injuries, boosted healing for issues like cold, fever etc, reduced blood pressure and lower chances of heart-attack (as per the American Heart Association).

To go further and get the best results, it is advised to practice mindfulness and meditation in conjunction with a daily exercise routine like running, yoga, sports etc.

Benefit #6 : Relationship Satisfaction.

In a Huffington Post article titled *How Mindfulness Can Save Your Relationship*, psychologist and author Lisa Firestone writes that mindfulness is a valuable tool for facing the challenges of staying connected to your partner. When couples get into a fight, their emotions start to spiral out of control and that results in resentment which can be considered the bedrock of most relationship failures. They start expressing themselves through the negative end of the emotional spectrum like hate, anger, pain etc.

So how does mindfulness help in getting our emotional breakdown under control and put a metaphorical lid on the outbursts? By being more aware of your state of mind and that of your partner, you don't react impulsively but take a moment to respond instead. This can be done by taking a few breaths and being in the moment instead of being flung away by your emotions. If you can be calmer in your interactions with your partner, it will lead to a better channel of communication. This can happen if either one of the people in the relationship is more aware and mindful. Once one of you starts being calmer, it is much easier for the other person to also get tuned to it and respond positively. It's no wonder when people say that relationships are like mirrors.

Other benefits of mindfulness include lower chance of depression, higher chance of overcoming addiction, memory boosts etc. It goes without saying that investing in learning and practicing mindfulness is worth every penny

Chapter 3

Techniques to Practice Mindfulness

In this chapter, we will cover 10 practical ways to train yourself to be more mindful. Please keep in mind that the goal of these exercises is to shift your attention and focus to the present moment. If you can achieve that somehow, the purpose of mindfulness is served.

As you read ahead, you might find yourself saying "But this is too simple to be effective". If you do, you must understand that there can only be so much instruction on how to be mindful. Eventually, it is you who must be aware and try to align your thoughts and emotions. The techniques described here will serve as mere guidelines for effective mindfulness.

Feel free to learn about each of the described techniques and pick those that you like best. Start with 2-5 minutes of a single technique and expand it to however long you want. You can change techniques based on your interest. Around 20 minutes of mindfulness per day will give you amazing results. It might take you a couple of days to notice the changes to your living condition and overall state of mind.

Technique #1 : Vipassanā

Vipassanā is a sanskrit term for Mindfulness Meditation. Needless to say, this is the most widespread and recommended technique of them all. The gist of it has been covered in chapter 1.

Mindfulness meditation is not a way of revamping your entire personality. Meditation does not change who you are. It just brings you closer to who you are naturally, by developing awareness. If you are happy, it makes you be aware of it. If you are sad, it brings your attention to it as well.

You might be wondering, "If I'm sad/angry and I'm more aware of the fact that I'm sad/angry, how does it help me?" Well, that's the magic of mindfulness meditation. By being aware of our emotions and going deeper into the present moment, we alleviate the suffering. We just exist. Pain and suffering are two different things. Pain is natural. But suffering is a choice. It occurs when we try to run away from our discomfort and pain but are unable to. By not trying to run away from pain but rather embracing it and being aware of it, the veils of suffering are lifted.

"The source of suffering is our attempt to escape from our direct experience."

\- Buddha

Step-1 : Pick your spot.

Find a room or an open place in your vicinity that has a calm environment. If you can dedicate a spot in your house or garden just for mindfulness meditation, that'd be great. You can even go fancy and decorate it with zen/buddhist covers, drapes, cushions, scented candles etc. Own your spot and make it homely so that you feel welcomed whenever you want to practice mindfulness.

Step-2 : Get into position.

Once you've fixed your spot, get into a sitting position. Make sure your hips are at a higher position than your knees. You can do this by either sitting on a chair or a cushion with your legs crossed. This is important because if you don't follow this, you won't be able to sit comfortably for long. Also make sure to keep your back(spine) straight vertically to avoid drowsiness. Taking support of a wall is fine. Relax and loosen your muscles to ensure they're not stiff and tight. Your hands can rest on your thighs, palms facing down.

Step-3 : Observer your breath.

Shift your focus on the movement of air in and out of your body. Do not force yourself or scold yourself for not maintaining attention. The key is to shift your focus towards your breath in a very subtle and gentle manner whenever you find it drifting. There should be no mental turbulence when you are shifting or maintaining focus. If you're a beginner, start with 5-10 minutes per day. I can't stress enough on the importance of making mindfulness meditation a habit. The toughest part about mindfulness is not the act of mindfulness itself but rather developing the discipline required to practice it everyday without fail. Try to set yourself up for a goal of 5 minutes of mindfulness meditation for atleast 10 days. 5 minutes is not really that big of a deal. Once you finish the 10-days goal, move it up to 10minutes per day for another 10 days. This is a practical and achievable method to developing the mindfulness habit.

Technique #2 : Urge Surfing

This is a technique developed by the late psychology professor Alan Marlatt in regards to addiction treatment. The concept is pretty simple. Think of an urge as a wave. When it hits, you have two choices. To struggle and sink or to relax and float. Just as waves are a natural part of the ocean, urges are a natural part of life. As a mindfulness practitioner, your goal is to ride out the wave without engaging with it. If you engage in battle with your urges, you cannot win. Even worse, you can give them more power. So the best thing to do is *keep calm and surf the urge.*

To practice this technique, sit in a quiet place and allow your attention to dwell on the areas of body where the urge hits. For example, if you get the urge of eating chocolate/candy, focus on the tongue, mouth watering sensation etc. Just be attentive to the bodily changes. It is important to note where exactly the urge originates from.

After identifying the region of the body where the urge is predominant, bring your attention to the details. What do the sensations feel like? Is there a tingling, warmth, pressure, pain? Get as specific as you can. Only by doing this can you understand, in entirety, the nature and effect of the urge on your body.

Next, momentarily shift your attention to your breath. Allow yourself to notice the body sensations in conjunction with the breath. If they are too strong, gently shift your focus back to them. Through out this process, you should be as gentle with your attention as possible. Notice how shifting the attention to the urges, changes their magnitude.

As we noted, every urge is like a wave. It rises and falls. So when you are paying attention to it, realize and anticipate the nullification of the urge. If it helps, you can say to yourself, "I'm just observing the rise and fall of the wave." The good news is that no matter how big the wave seems to be, if you are patient enough to breathe, watch and observe, sooner or later it will fall and you can ride it out.

Bonus Tip : Being detached and observant of the urge is understandably tough in the beginning. So if you're struggling to pay attention without loosing control, you can become active in being mindful. Describe the sensation in words, say it out loud, draw references and examples to explain it. Anything you can do to sustain attention will give you an edge over the urge. Happy Surfing !

Technique #3 : Group-based Mindfulness training

With the right number of enthusiastic people, this technique can give you the best results in the shortest time span. There is also evidence that shows that group-based mindfulness is as effective as CBT(Cognitive Behavioral Therapy).

You can either join or create a mindfulness focus group or club and try various fun activities. This is also useful in reducing social anxiety. Here are some activities you can try with a group :

- Play two truths and a lie. Every person has to say 3 things about themselves out of which 2 are true and 1 is false. All the others guess which of the 3 statements is false and explain why they felt so. This practice not only helps you be mindful of the other person's statements but also improves your person-reading skills as you have to be mindful and aware of the gestures, signs, tone of voice etc.

- Do a guided meditation with or without audio (e.g, binaural beats, tara brach's summer smile meditation track, Headspace app).

- Go on a group walk at the beach, park, woods etc. As you're moving through the environment, try to notice the sounds of nature, the smells, the color of the sky, leaves, ground etc. And later you can each express what you were able to observe and be aware of.

Technique #4 : The Raisin Exercise

This technique is famous among many mindfulness and meditation groups. It is quite similar in concept to *The Heart of the Rose* technique described by Robin Sharma in his book *The Monk who sold his Ferrari*.

The raisin method goes as follows. First, you take a raisin and hold it between your fingers or on the palm. Look at it from all possible angles. Develop an insatiable curiosity towards the raisin. Observe the texture, the density, the size, the strength, the elasticity and everything else about it. Use all your senses in this observation. Note the smell. What does the smell make you feel? What does it remind you of? Now put the raisin on your tongue and observe the taste and feel of it in your mouth. Take your time and explore everything. And then swallow it and pay attention to it as it travels down to your stomach to become a part of you.

The fundamental idea behind this technique is to take in as many details about the raisin as possible. By doing so, you shift your total undivided attention towards the raisin which encapsulates "the present moment" for you. This can actually be done with any object like a leaf, pen etc. The reason for taking raisin as an example is to involve the sense of taste as well.

Technique #5 : The Body Scan

This particular technique has been found to help people in healing themselves over time without the need of any particular tools or medicines.

Begin by lying on your back comfortably with your palms facing up. Alternatively, you can sit on a chair keeping your back straight. Relax your muscles and let your entire body become still.

Start bringing your attention to every body part and organ from the crown of your head to the toes of your feet. Be conscious about every movement, every tingle, every pressure point. While you scan your body, do not attempt to force anything. Just observe as if you were watching your body from the outside.

Once you're done with a full single body attention sweep, repeat it back from the head to the feet for a couple of more times. After that, with 2 breaths, gently bring your attention back to the environment. Start noticing your surroundings and let yourself wake up with full energy. With some practice, you will be able to identify the regions of your body which feel a bit dysfunctional and pay attention to them using this technique. Advanced practitioners will be able to recognize and locate health issues in their body before they become serious.

Technique #6 : The Five Senses Exercise

This is a relatively simple technique which you can do almost anywhere. The basic idea is to be aware of the objects you are currently experiencing through your 5 senses.

Sight : Observe 5 things you can see in your environment, one at a time. These can be anything non-living like rocks, buildings, water etc or living creatures like birds, squirrels, dogs, cats or even humans and crowds (don't get yourself in trouble by staring though).

Taste : You can practice this while eating your food or at the least, you can try drinking a glass of water or eating a piece of fruit. Notice as your taste buds fire up and the saliva starts getting mixed in your mouth.

Touch : Here's a fun fact. Your skin is lined up with a specialized layer of *tactile cells* which help you sense the feeling of touch and pressure. But over time, they stop responding to similar stimuli. That is why our feeling of the clothes decreases after we wear them. So this is a great opportunity to revive that feeling and pay attention to all the things touching your skin like your clothes, ring, watch, shoes, the wind, the ground etc.

Smell : According to nature.com and other science studies, the human nose can detect around 1 trillion odors! So put this brilliant organ to use and try to filter out different scents. How do they feel? Pleasant or Foul? The more you practice the more you develop your sense of smell.

Hearing : This is something I personally practice every morning and has been very effective as a mindfulness technique. I go to a park or the beach or some place away from heavy noise like traffic, construction etc. After getting to a relatively calm state of mind, I listen to all the sounds that my ears catch like bird chirps, water and waves, the trees and grass being blown by the wind etc. After 10 mins of practicing this, you feel very calm, peaceful and close to nature.

Technique #7 : Self-Enquiry based Meditation

Sri Ramana Maharshi, a revered Indian sage and spiritual teacher, is famous for his recommendation and endorsement of this technique. As Ramana Maharshi put it, the key to liberation and enlightenment is to have an effortless awareness of being which can be acquired by constantly chasing the identify (the " I ") of your thoughts. Here are some example questions you can ask yourself during the practice of self-enquiry :

- Who am I ?

- What does it feel to be me ?

- Where is this sense of "I" and "me" coming from ?

The goal of self-enquiry is to identify your "Self" or the source of your consciousness. In the words of late Ramana Maharshi, "You are awareness. Since you are awareness, there is no need to attain or cultivate it. If one gives up being aware of the non-self then only pure awareness remains, and that is the Self."

There is no supposed time of the day to practice self-enquiry. It can be done at any point of time and is actually recommended by some gurus to practice it through out your waking hours. But if you are someone with a job, a family, living in a city/town with work to do, you may find constant self-enquiry annoying and unfruitful. In that case, limit it to your free-time off from work at your home away from all the buzz.

Technique #8 : The 5-minute Bell Exercise

This technique can be performed in groups or in classrooms for kids. The idea is pretty straight forward. You take the help of a bell (or any timed sound effect for that matter) that rings every 2 minutes to align your attention with the present moment. If you find yourself distracted, it acts as a reminder to bring your focus back. If you're not, it can act as the object of your focus i.e, being aware of the sound as it rings and fades away.

You can use guided meditation audio or mobile apps if you can't find a group willing to take part in this exercise. There are a lot of "meditation timer" and "mindfulness bell" apps available for the android and apple platforms.

Just like the Pavlov's dogs in his classical conditioning experiment, you will be trained to let go of all your mental clutter and focus on your breath and the present moment when you hear the bell. You can increase the time interval between the bell rings as you progress in your mindfulness practice and become more efficient at maintaining concentration.

Technique #9 : R.A.I.N

This is more of a process than a specific technique. Made popular by Tara Brach, a leading psychologist and teacher in the field of meditation and spirituality, R.A.I.N is an acronym to describe the mindfulness process. Although it can be used by anybody in any state of mind, it is usually followed by recovering addicts or people struggling with difficult negative emotions like sadness and suffering.

R – Recognize

This is the first step to almost any emotional healing. The realization that a problem exists and the identification of it. You can ask questions like "What exactly is going on inside me?" Recognizing problems correctly is a mature way to go about life and growth. It involves self-reflection and contemplation or discussion with others. Just consider the assumptions and believes you currently hold and one by one, flip them and see if there seems to be any truth to your reality. If not then that belief is probably obsolete. Try this if you're a beginner and have trouble recognizing your problem.

A – Accept

This can be really hard if the problem you've recognized is either very critical or seems irrelevant. For example, in the book Steve Jobs by Walter Isaacson, although jobs was diagnosed with cancer, he avoided medical treatment for a lot of days. This made the issue worse and he later regretted it. Accepting the problem can be a rather unpleasant experience because it hurts your ego. And nobody likes being vulnerable or weak. But make no mistake, this is a very important step in recovery.

I – Investigate

Once you've accepted your problem, you need to develop a curiosity to find a solution for it. Explore how you're feeling in your body and mind. Pay attention to the thoughts and the body sensations. This is where you get the full effect of mindfulness. Treat yourself like a baby and ask gentle and soothing questions. Open up to yourself, be honest and true to yourself. This means you have to create a feeling of safety and security for your inner self.

N – Non-Identification

Once you have found the reason for the problem, your next step is to make the problem go away. But with emotional problems, it's not as easy as it sounds. A head-on approach doesn't always work when it comes to matters of the mind. Around 95% of our brain belongs to the unconscious and subconscious which we have no direct control over. Since this is where our emotions come from, we have to realize that as a conscious being, we do not have complete control over our emotions. This will lead to a separation of awareness where you are detached from your thoughts and emotions. This is the final phase of suffering. And the beginning phase of recovery.

Technique #10 : Other Informal Techniques

Exercise : In his best selling book *Tools of Titans*, author Tim Ferris points out that a common pattern among self made billionaires and high achievers is some form of mindfulness practice every morning. For example, Arnold Schwarzenegger, the body-builder, actor, California governor (among other things), uses physical training as a form of mindfulness and meditation. Exercise gives you numerous health benefits and also, because of the pain involved, forces you to stay in the present moment. You can start with running daily for 10mins.

Mindful Eating : Just like the raisin technique, you can try paying attention to what you're eating through out your day. Habits like slow-eating and being mindful of what you're eating (e.g, veganism) have been shown to lead to better digestion, higher energy levels and lower chance of obesity. Besides, wouldn't you like to actually enjoy the taste and feel of your food instead of just gulping it down?

Music : There are a lot of audio playlists you can find on the internet for help with guided mindfulness and meditation. For example, certain binaural beats, which are generated by mixing audio frequencies, can help you get to a more relaxed state of consciousness. You can sit in a comfortable position and listen to any of the audio clips while maintaining focus on your breath.

Staring at a Candle : This was taught to me by my yoga teacher a couple of years ago. Here's what you need to do. Go to a calm space, turn of all lights and make it totally dark. Sit in a comfortable position and light a candle in front of you. Start by focusing on the tip of the flame and slowly extend it to the body of the flame, the thread, the wax, the whole candle. Expand your awareness of the candle until you perceive it as one object. After that, expand your observation radius slowly, starting with the space near the candle, and then a bit farther and so on until you have awareness of the entire room.

Chapter 4

Cultivating Mindfulness
into daily life

Sustained practice of mindfulness is what brings the greatest results. To get them, you have to incorporate mindfulness as a habit in your day-to-day life. You need to make a plan and stick to it. In this chapter, you will learn tips and tricks that can be used to develop a daily habit of mindfulness.

Tip #1 : The Power of the Morning Ritual

Morning time just after waking up is when your mind is least cluttered with thoughts and emotions. Brain scans of various people have shown that the pre-frontal cortex of the brain, which is responsible for focus and attention, is most active just after waking up. This is because during sleep, our memories and learnings are consolidated into the deeper neural network of our brain which frees up the cortex for fresh processing.

So why not practice mindfulness when you are most likely to get the best results? Also, you are least distracted just after waking up. This is an advantage. As they say, if you win the morning, you win the whole day. So it makes sense to set your day up for success by finishing off the mindfulness routine first thing in the morning.

Tip #2 : Keep it Short and Sweet

The toughest part of building a habit is the initial phase where you struggle to change your state of mind from "I don't feel like doing it" to "I want to do it now". He who can motivate himself to do what is required will have the easiest time building the habit and also in life in general. This begs the question "How do you go from not wanting to do it to wanting to do it?". Let us find an answer to this question by trying to reverse-engineer the desired state of mind. What makes us want to do something inherently boring and hard?

The answer lies in the question itself. We don't want to do anything that is boring and hard. So if you can figure out a way to make it easy and exciting, you will have better time developing the habit. Easy and Exciting – that's just another phrase for Short and Sweet. So what you want to do is start with just 5 minutes of mindfulness per day for 10 days. And don't worry about whether you were able to achieve a Zen-like state of pure consciousness while you practice it. Lower your expectations as much as possible. Redefine success as spending those 5 minutes in an **attempt** for mindfulness.

With this framework, you will feel success everyday and that leads to a positive reinforcement to your brain and you will start liking mindfulness more. And that leads to you practicing mindfulness more. And that leads to more positive reinforcement. So it becomes a healthy positive loop of actions and rewards whose outcome is a well developed habit of mindfulness.

Tip #3 : Create Effective Cues

Humans are creatures of habit. No matter how disciplined you are, without an effective system in place that helps you loop into the habit and track your progress, you will eventually fall out of the habit. So it is important to have cues spread out through your home and work place to trigger you into the required state of mind. These cues can be anything from sticky notes and alarms to having a personal trainer or guide/mentor. Here are some examples of effective cues.

<u>Time of the day</u> : You do not need to remind yourself to brush in the morning every day because at an unconscious level, you have associated morning time with brushing teeth. So start practicing mindfulness immediately after brushing your teeth in the morning and it will become a habit set in stone because everyday you will brush your teeth and that implies that everyday you will practice mindfulness.

<u>Calendar Notifications</u> : This is pretty straightforward. Plan your days, weeks and months on your calendar. Set specific deadlines and reminders. For example, you can have a reminder that pops up at 11am, 4pm and 9pm every day that will remind you to practice the habit for 5mins. I have used this to develop good habits like drinking water, meditation, writing, exercise etc.

<u>Set up Accountability</u> : By informing your friends/family that you're taking up mindfulness as a daily habit, you set yourself up for social accountability which has been shown to be very effective in developing and maintaining habits. You will experience healthy social/peer pressure to practice the habit daily and also get cues that will keep you on your toes. If you feel that your friends or family might not like to remind you of your habit, you can join a mindfulness or meditation club. The good thing about these clubs/groups is that everybody is on the same boat as you. Everyone wants to develop the mindfulness habit. So it will be easier to find accountability buddies. In the worst case scenario, you can just enforce a self-constraint that whenever you miss the 5min mindfulness practice during the

day, you will do 10 pushups. What this does is associate pain with not practicing mindfulness so the next time you get a reminder, your brain will naturally be inclined towards doing the mindfulness activity instead of experiencing pain. Thank God for mental conditioning, eh?

Tip #4 : Weave it into existing routines

The more you practice mindfulness, the better your mental health will become. So you need to find every excuse you can to practice mindfulness during the waking hours. You can even do this while waiting in line or getting stuck in traffic. Try to find a way to mix mindfulness with a pre-existing habit or routine like cooking, walking the dog, bathing etc. Any amount of time you can spare will benefit you. The good news is that since you already follow these existing habits, putting a little extra effort is not that big of a deal. Plus, you will be leveraging the existing mental framework associated with the old habit to form a new habit. Isn't that smart?

Before we dive into the next tip, I just want to say that I hope you're enjoying the read. I've spent a lot of time doing the required research and learning to share this message on mindfulness with you. So if you like it, please <u>leave a review on Amazon</u>. It would help a lot. Thanks.

Tip #5 : Cut Down Options

Decision-making sucks up your mental resources. If you wake up everyday and debate with yourself on whether you need to do it or not then you probably won't. You shouldn't have to decide. You should just fall into the process of it. For example, Barack Obama insisted that while he was in office, he would wear only black, blue and gray suits. "I shouldn't have to decide on what I'm going to wear everyday as I already have too many decisions to make for the country." he said.

In the best-seller *Predictably Irrational*, author Dan Ariely points out that keeping doors open actually prohibits us from taking action in a specific direction. So he encourages people to voluntarily close certain options. This will supposedly help us de-paralyze ourselves in the process of decision-making and action-taking.

So how can you apply this to mindfulness? Make sure that in your dedicated time slot for practicing mindfulness (create one if you haven't already), stay away from your mobile phone, social media, notifications, distractions etc. This way, you can't be reminded of events that require your immediate attention. In order to develop a long-term habit of mindfulness, you need to let go of the short-term attention seeking activities and events. This is not to say that you shouldn't respond to emergencies but that you should delay distractions and build up the habit of mindfulness until it becomes second nature to you.

Chapter 5

How to Increase Focus

with Mindfulness

Let's start by trying to understand what focus actually is. Focus can be generally defined as the act of paying attention to what is necessary (important) while avoiding what is unnecessary (unimportant). In this chapter, we will look at focus in the context of our day-to-day mental activities (more commonly known as "work"). We will get a glance of what it feels like to have complete focus, how it can improve our lives, some of the common reasons people lose focus and finally, how mindfulness can help improve our focus levels.

<u>What a focused mind feels like</u>

Have you ever seen a laser in real life? A proper laser can emit light so focused that it can cut through solid steel! On the other hand, a bulb also emits light but can hardly burn anything, much

49

less cut through steel. This is the difference between a focused mind and a distracted mind.

A focused mind has the ability to process information, filter out unnecessary options and get to the goal in the fastest route possible. It is very similar to the phenomenon of "flow" or "tunnel vision" or "being in the zone".

"The average human looks without seeing, listens without hearing, touches without feeling, eats without tasting, inhales without smelling, and talks without thinking."

\- Leonardo da Vinci

Benefits Of Having Focus

I don't think you need to be sold on the importance of having focus. If you are already convinced about this, I suggest you skip to the next section. However, if you're curious about what practical benefits focus can bring to your life, here are a few you can get by building a ninja-like focus.

Benefit #1 : You will get things done faster. Obviously we're referring to the mental tasks and activities that you need to finish with your brain. Improving focus might not increase your deadlift capacity. But if you put in the time and effort to develop focus, you will slowly start noticing something strange. Other people tend to take much longer time to finish the same tasks than you. Also, what seems easy to you will appear like a mammoth task to them.

"People think it's fun to be a super genius, but they don't realize how hard it is to put up with all the idiots."

- Bill Watterson (author of Calvin and Hobbes)

Benefit #2 : You will get better at problem solving. Human progress is measured by the scale of problems we are able to solve. The ancient man was able to solve the problem of food and staying warm. In the modern age, we have solved the problem of gravity i.e, going to the moon and beyond. All of this happened because we honed our problem solving skills. With increased focus, you will be able to objectively define the problem, identify the issue and filter out irrelevant fixes to end up at the right solution. This process involves a lot of critical analysis and paying attention to what is required and ignoring what's not. Notice how this is precisely what focus is about, according to our stated definition.

Benefit #3 : You will feel more positive. Getting more work done and possessing the ability to control your attention will make you happier. Nobody likes being distracted. Even more so when we know that we're supposed to be working on our tasks. By developing focus, not only can you finish your tasks faster, but you will also feel better for being able to evade and avoid distractions like a pro. This creates a positive feedback loop where you feel good for staying focused which develops your ability to stay focused which in turn makes you feel even better.

<u>Why we loose focus</u>

Attention is a depleting mental resource. There can be a lot of reasons for losing focus depending on your psychology and circumstances. Listed below are 2 of the most common reasons for losing focus in our day-to-day life.

Reason #1 : Distractions

Studies have shown that will power and focus are actually finite resources. This means that the more distracted you are, the tougher it is to get your focus back. This is especially true in the current age of internet and social media. According to an article by Daniel Levitin from *The Guardian*, research of a former visiting professor of psychology has found that trying to concentrate on a task when an unread email is sitting in your inbox can reduce your effective IQ by 10 points. This goes to show that being exposed to distractions and social media in particular can be detrimental to our brain's performance when it comes to cognitively demanding tasks.

In his book *Deep Work,* author Cal Newport writes that the ability to focus on hard tasks is becoming increasingly rare and valuable at the same time. This means that the people who can figure out how to develop and maintain focus amidst the distractions will thrive in our economy.

Reason #2 : Lack of energy

We have all experienced this. You can rarely focus on work when you're exhausted physically and/or mentally. Your brain needs high levels of oxygen and fuel to get the energy it needs to function properly. Although you can develop and maintain focus while being unhealthy, the best results are obtained when your body is physically fit. They don't say *"A sound mind in a sound body"* for nothing. A healthy body will produce the right levels of hormones to balance the stress of mental wear out. From personal experience, I can say that being physically fit by doing regular exercise has given me a natural boost in productivity and my ability to focus. In the book *The Power of Full Engagement*, authors Jim and Tony point out that the key to peak performance(both physical and mental) is energy management. High achievers balance energy expenditure with intermittent energy renewal through optimal relaxation. It pays to learn how to invest your energy well.

So if you are able to spike your energy levels and avoid distractions, you will find that the intensity and duration of your focus increase rapidly.

How exactly Mindfulness can build your Focus

We have already understood that being distracted is one of the biggest reasons for losing focus. If you can eliminate distractions to your brain, you have effectively won half the battle. Here is how mindfulness can help you avoid and deal with distractions.

Think of your attention as a muscle. The more you train it, the better it gets. When you're being mindful, you practice living in the present moment. That means you're training your brain's neural network to prioritize paying attention to the current moment over the past or future(distractions). By repeatedly bringing your attention back to the present moment, you get good at avoiding distractions. The more mindful you are, the more focused you are on the present moment. This is in line with the definition of focus which is paying attention to the important and avoiding the unimportant.

Once you get good at mindfulness, you can translate that developed focus into any field. This is because you are still paying attention to the present moment but just different forms of it. Instead of paying attention to your breath, you will be paying attention to the object of work like a book or a presentation or a software.

A paper published in *Psychiatry Research NeuroImaging* Journal has shown that practicing mindfulness meditation leads to increase in the brain's gray matter density. For the unaware, gray matter is the part of the brain that handles various functions such as sensory perception, self-control, decision making etc. People with denser gray matter can learn better, memorize faster and most importantly, maintain focus on important tasks for much longer duration.

<u>Bonus tips to increase Focus</u>

Bonus Tip #1 : Chew gum. Seriously. As mentioned on a podcast by Scientific American, chewing gum increases oxygen flow to your brain and also injects some insulin into your blood resulting in higher focus.

Bonus Tip #2 : Find a line of work that is both interesting and important to you. This has to be genuinely passionate for you and demand your undivided attention. Otherwise, your brain activates a *default network* that switches your attention to other stimuli.

Bonus Tip #3 : No more multi-tasking. One task at a time, fellas. In reality our brain cannot pay attention to more than one thing at a time. So people who think they are multi-tasking are actually switching their attention between different tasks rapidly. This has been shown to fray your brain out and reduce productivity levels.

Bonus Tip #4 : Observe your body's natural energy rhythm and align your work accordingly. Your brain is usually very active just after breakfast and at dusk. So schedule your heavy-lifting tasks during those times and maybe take a power-nap or go for a walk during the afternoon. Also don't forget to take breaks in between work sessions, get ample sleep, eat nutritious food and exercise regularly for best results.

Chapter 6

Finding Inner Peace and Happiness

Do you feel a nagging sensation in your life? Is there something lacking? Chances are you probably do not have inner peace if you answered Yes. People who have inner peace do not complain. But there's no need to fret if you do. We'll discuss ideas in this chapter that will give you a perspective on inner peace, how that can lead to happiness and how to get there through the practice of mindfulness.

Ego says, "Once everything falls into place, I'll have peace." Spirit says, "Find peace and everything will fall into place."

\- Marianne Williamson

The Essence of Inner Peace

Gautama Buddha said that *Nirvana* is the ultimate goal of life.

The term *Nirvana* comes from Sanskrit and is used to describe a state of peaceful existence that is independent of external or internal stimuli. According to religions like Buddhism and Hinduism, Nirvana is true liberation and leads to freedom from suffering.

Inner Peace is almost synonymous with contentment. It's like having your inner jar of needs completely filled. There cannot be inner peace when there is a burning thirst to be quenched. Joy and happiness are outcomes of that state of mind called *Inner Peace*.

Inner Turmoil is the opposite of Inner Peace. Although there can be different reasons for that turmoil, many people loose inner peace by wanting to be something but later realizing that they cannot. How does one overcome that kind of limitations? The answer is...through self-acceptance. When you own your flaws, you will be one with yourself and that inner pain of not being something you're not will cease to exist.

"Never forget who you are. The rest of the world will not. Wear it like armor and it can't be used to hurt you."

\- Tyrion Lannister from Game of Thrones

Inner Peace is more about being than doing. But as far as doing goes, the act of forgiveness will go a long way to help you in self-acceptance. As you go on life's journey, you will have many experiences and face many situations where you don't like who you are or how you reacted or how you feel or think. This is quite normal. The important thing to do is be aware of what you are, what you like about yourself and don't. Once you get a better understanding of your personality through contemplation, you can start the self-healing process of forgiving yourself for your mistakes, bad decisions and character flaws.

Another great tool for getting rid of your inner turmoil is Gratitude. When you are grateful for what you have and what life has to offer, your outlook changes. Instead of complaining about problems, you will inject positivity into your daily experiences. At a physiological level, you cannot be grateful and feel anger or fear at the same time.

The bottom line is that inner turmoil occurs when our thoughts/emotions effect us negatively. The essence of inner peace lies in realizing that you are not your thoughts/emotions. The practice of mindfulness teaches you to be aware and pay attention to what goes on in your head. This will create the gap that is needed between you and your thoughts/emotions. As you are mindful and separate yourself from your thoughts/emotions, you will tend to be less effected by them. This detachment is the gateway to inner peace.

<u>How happiness will result from inner peace.</u>

"Happiness is not a goal. It's a byproduct."

\- Eleanor Roosevelt

There is a fundamental difference in how happiness is perceived between the western school of thought and the eastern. People in the west typically tend to believe that they will be happy when they achieve their goals and acquire material possessions like money, cars, muscles, mansions etc. The eastern philosophy preaches that happiness is not about the external but rather the internal. That sustainable long-term happiness comes when we are at peace with ourselves without any inner conflicts.

Happiness is an outcome of our attitude. If you are calm on the inside, you can feel happy no matter how chaotic the external world is. The famous movie *Life is Beautiful* depicts exactly this philosophy.

Please note that inner peace and happiness are two different states of mind. Just because you have no worries, it doesn't mean that you have happiness. To put it another way, having no negatives doesn't correlate with having a positive. Unlike inner peace, which is about being, happiness is more of an active process. To feel happy, you need to do stuff that makes you happy. It is important to understand what sort of stuff makes you happy over the long term. Too often, people look for happiness in the wrong places. An online course by UC Berkley, called *The Science of Happiness*, teaches that a major reason for happiness lies in relationships and social life. Having a purpose and serving others are two of the best ways to lead a happy life.

How Mindfulness can help

As we have seen, detachment from thoughts and emotions is a great way to eliminate suffering and attain inner peace. As you maintain your distance from the emotions that try to grab your attention, you will be less influenced by the drama they try to create. This will inevitably result in a more peaceful state of being.

Letting go of the desire to control is another great way to have inner peace. When you practice mindfulness, you surrender yourself to the present moment. You become just an observer. This can be very liberating. You are not burdened by any need to control situations or people. You just let the chips fall where they may. This also translates to lower stress & anxiety.

In chapter-2, we talked about how Self-Awareness is one of the major benefits of Mindfulness. Self-awareness is the stepping stone for Self-acceptance. That's because you can't accept yourself if you don't understand yourself. By practicing mindfulness daily for 10-30min, you pay attention to your inner mental banter which tells you who you really are. When you start observing your thoughts from an outsider's perspective, you get a better picture of what you like, what you don't like, what you care about etc. These nuances will help you get a picture of your own character and personality. Once you truly understand who you are, you can appreciate the beauty of being you. And that's how you eliminate insecurities and finally accept yourself. May the peace be with you :)

Chapter 7

Destroy Stress & Anxiety

Why we feel Stress

Stress is a natural phenomenon caused by the body in response to events that are perceived as harmful or threatening. This perception of danger is not always conscious. For example, when you suddenly see a Tiger across the road, your body's defense system is automatically activated, releasing large amounts of stress hormones, cortisol and adrenaline, into your blood stream. Your heart rate and blood pressure get spiked, muscles become tense, breathing gets faster and your senses are elevated. All of this is an involuntary response called "Fight or Flight" where your body prepares you to either fight the threat(in this case, a Tiger) or run away from it.

As you can guess, not all stress is bad. In fact, if it weren't for stress, we wouldn't be alive. This is not to say that all kinds of stress are positive. When stress occurs in an unguided manner and in heavy doses, it can lead to a lot of health issues(both physical and mental).

Stress in animals tends to be episodic while in humans it tends to be chronic. Chronic stress will keep the levels of cortisol always high in your body. This results in all kinds of issues like high blood sugar, obesity and muscle breakdown. Animals don't have stress issues because they go by their instinct. That is another way of saying that they live in the moment. If you are interested and want to read up on this further, check out the famous book *Why Zebras don't have Ulcers* by Stanford Biologist Robert Sapolsky.

How to Eliminate Stress with Mindfulness

There is a difference between response and reaction. The difference is that a response is generated after thinking and processing the stimulus whereas a reaction is impulsive. Mindfulness can help you become more responsive instead of reactive.

"Mindfulness is a pause – the space between stimulus and response. That's where choice lies."

- Tara Brach

People who experience and understand stress will know that everyone has unique stress triggers and stress reactions. The stress triggers occur when the subject feels a harm or threat to their survival at a subliminal level. To relieve this stress and deflate the threat, a stress response is generated. And the stress response varies among individuals. For some it is eating junk food or drugs or gambling while for others it is exercise or spending time with their family or pets. A healthy stress response will build your personality and make you stronger.

What mindfulness does is build a gap between the stress trigger and stress response. This gives you more time to analyze the situation, cool down and choose the right response. Instead of doing the bad things in a haste, you will be more inclined to normalize the stress by looking at the situation objectively.

It has also been found that practicing mindfulness will reduce neural activity in a part of your brain called the Amygdala. It is responsible for identifying threats in the environment and hijack our cortex(responsible for critical thinking) if there is any possibility of danger. Sadly, the hypersensitivity of amygdala results in too many stress triggers and immediate stress responses. So mindfulness can actually help you turn the amygdala's intervention down a notch and experience lesser stress.

Mindfulness Trick for Handling Stress

Whenever you feel stress again, take 10mins off, sit in a quiet place and practice any of the mindfulness techniques covered in chapter-3. What you want to do is remember and imagine vividly the situation that triggered your stress. Since stress is a physiological phenomenon, you can pay attention to the various body parts, sensations and feelings that are changing because of the stress. Pay close attention and try to precisely spot the emotion that is responsible for the stress. Be mindful of the emotion and what it does to your body. Try to feel the changes in your body in conjunction with breathing and relaxation. If you can, put your hand on the location of your body which feels effected and gently massage it with a sense of compassion and care. With enough practice, you should be able to not only handle stress but avoid it altogether by developing stress resistance.

Chapter 8

Conclusion

We have gone through many concepts in this book that give a basic understanding of mindfulness and the philosophy behind it. If you've paid attention, you will be in possession of knowledge about various mindfulness techniques, tips to develop a daily habit out of it, the essence of inner peace and how to use mindfulness to improve your focus. These are just some of the things we've gone through in this book. If you feel like you might have missed something, don't worry. Here's a quick recap of what we learned.

Summary

- Mindfulness can be defined as being aware of the inside(thoughts, emotions) and outside(environment, other beings).

- Mindfulness is medicine for the body and soul. It helps in overcoming addictions and identifying issues in the body.

- Research from various neurological studies has highlighted the huge upsides of practicing mindfulness. For example, an increase in empathy, higher focus, higher happiness levels, better response to various therapies.

- Other benefits of mindfulness include self-awareness, stress reduction and prevention, emotional regulation, better relationships and overall health.

- The most common technique to practice mindfulness is Vipassanā which involves paying attention to the breath initially and then extending it to become a passive observation of thoughts and emotions.

- Other techniques like the body scan and raisin exercise are also popular.

- The easiest way to develop the habit of mindfulness is to practice it early in the morning immediately after waking up and getting ready.

- It is important to not put pressure on yourself while trying to maintain attention during mindfulness. Starting small is also a good idea for beginners.

- Focus is nothing but paying attention to what is important and ignoring what is not.

- By practicing mindfulness, you develop the attention muscle and your control over it. This improves your focus and ability to ignore distractions.

- Other tips to increase focus are : chewing gum, avoiding multi-tasking and regular exercise.

- Inner Peace is a state of mind that can be reached using mindfulness. Self-acceptance plays a huge role in having inner peace.

- Detachment(temporary) from thoughts and emotions is also good way to attain inner peace.

- Stress is a natural phenomenon. It occurs when we feel threatened by a danger. Prolonged stress is very bad for physical and mental health.

- Mindfulness helps reduce stress because it creates a delay between the stress-trigger and the stress-response.

- It also reduces neural activity in the amygdala which leads to fewer impulsive stress responses.

- Whenever you feel anxious or stressed, notice how it affects your body and pay attention to the parts that have changed. By observing the changes in your body, you not only ground yourself but also develop stress resistance.

Did you like it?

This was my honest attempt to share my knowledge and to hopefully get you interested on the topic of Mindfulness. I truly believe that Mindfulness and Meditation hold the key to a peaceful, focused, happy life in this distracted world.

I want to thank you from the bottom of my heart for purchasing this book. I hope you found some value in the topics covered.

If you liked it, please <u>leave a review on Amazon</u> and let me know how you felt and what else you're interested in.

Want More ?

If you are into this kind of stuff like I am, then you need to join my list. Check out the link below for some amazing stuff on mindfulness, meditation, yoga, buddhism, zen, spirituality, personal development etc. I am constantly going through learning experiences and mentorship from some really great people(both online and offline). I want to share those insights and useful resources with you.

http://bit.ly/spirituality-and-stuff

Thanks again for taking your time out to read this. I hope you enjoyed the book and found some value.

Until next time,

Dharma Hazari.

Made in the USA
Columbia, SC
02 April 2018